SWITCHING TO YOUTH

SOUMYADEB BATABYAL

Copyright © Soumyadeb Batabyal
All Rights Reserved.

“I am committing this work of mine to my folks.”

Contents

Preface

Since childhood, I have run over a number of scientific writings. They are incredible and a little perplexing. A scientific writing is a report-cum-story that describes original research findings in a less detailed but more comprehensive way. The goal is to communicate the results of scientific study to others. To impart, science stories ought to be clear, compact, and efficient. In scientific writing, good language and grammar must be used to convey meaning in the fewest possible words. Coincidentally, I truly concede that it is far from simple or easy in actuality. You should contend on this point that those aforementioned assertions couldn't be disseminated among people in a simple manner. This book, "SWITCHING TO YOUTH", is an approach, you may say, bound to recount certain anecdotes about our ageing. Is it true or not that you are insane? Indeed, you may also express this to me. I found it remarkably captivating and felt a smidgen more insanity while composing this book. This work of mine most likely gives an intuitive grasp of ageing.

What occurs in our bodies when we age? What are the atomic and cell components that control ageing, and would we be able to postpone ageing by focusing on these cycles? We are on the whole mindful of the outer highlights that show up at advanced age, like kinks and silver hair however for what reason do we age and what precisely occurs inside our body when we age is considerably less perceived.

The mechanisms that contribute to the ageing process are a hot topic among researchers. However, it is commonly known that the functional decline associated with old age is caused by damage to genetic information, cells, and tissues that accumulate with age and cannot be restored by the body. But it's less apparent what causes this molecular damage and why it can be healed in young creatures but not in old ones. However, this book has been qualified to exhibit parts of anti-ageing and the ways of accomplishing it.

Acknowledgements

Composing a book is more fun than I suspected it would be and more remunerating than I might at any point have envisioned. No part of this would have been conceivable without Triparna, one of my dearest companions. While I was occupied with composing this book, she remained by my side and assisted me with the assets. She was as vital to this book's finishing as I was. Having a thought and transforming it into a book is just as hard as it sounds. The experience is both enlightening and fulfilling. I particularly need to thank the people that assisted in making this occur. Complete thanks to Notion Press.

Switching to Youth

CHAPTER ONE

INTRODUCTION

Hello there... I think you are now mindful of why you have arrived. You have, by certain means, ended up knowing specific things about your age. Clearly, we are not undying. At one point on schedule, we go downhill, become sluggish, foster sicknesses, and, in the end, kick the bucket. It is sure to happen to everyone. We as a whole get it and frequently wonder, "Imagine a scenario where things didn't work thusly?" What if we could dial back the clock and even turn it back to when we were young? All things considered, research has a slight edge in getting it going, in some measure theoretically and somewhat practically also. Research has emerged in developing some tools to programme our bodies in such a way that they could gain some strategies to achieve reverse ageing. Let's have a look at what this book has to offer.

Let's have a look at some of the aspects of health rejuvenation. Are you familiar with stem cells? What can I explain in simple terms? Let's suppose stem cells are cells that have the ability to develop into any sort of cell. Pluripotent cells have a high capacity for self-renewal and are frequently referred to as such. There's a growing body of data that suggests the ageing process can harm stem cells. The ability of stem cells to regenerate and specialize into different cell types deteriorates as they age. As a result, it's possible that ageing-induced declines in stem cell capabilities have a role in ageing-related ailments.

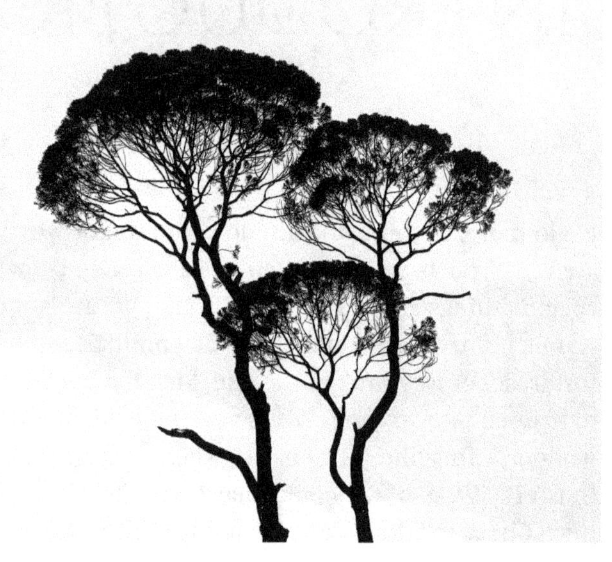

Let me take an example from the Sinclair Lab. They have developed ICE mice by inducing gene breaks that cause epigenetic changes accelerating ageing. They compared them to control mice that were at the same age as they are, *i.e.,* 16 months. According to them, "If DNA is the digital information on a compact disc, then ageing is due to scratches. We are searching for the polish. Our work has led us to identify reprogramming factors that we believe will enable us to reset a cell's epigenetic status and reverse its age". Nonetheless, after carrying out the aforesaid experiment, they came to the conclusion that the ICE mice had aged significantly faster than the control mice (normal). They were able to cause some DNA degradation in mice, causing them to age more quickly.

And do you know? DNA methylation could also take part in age determination. Scientists could tell your age by examining how much-methylated cytosine content you have from your mouth swab or from your blood sample. For much simplicity, you can say that you have aged much as you have a greater amount of methylated cytosine content.

Assuming you go through it exhaustively, a few things may come to you as minimally befuddling. Do you realise you can make your biological age fall behind your chronological age? The thing is you simply need to make significant epigenetic changes to your genome to qualify. Congratulation! You are green to go with the epigenetic clock, which has at long last been dialled back. Now you may be wondering, "Is it really that simple? What's more, the response was "no." I will be coming to shield my response in one minute. Before that, let me get straight to the point about specific things.

Battling against disease is additionally an incredible benefit for youngsters since this capacity weakens over the long haul. The thymus is one of the most urgent organs on the grounds that here, white blood cells are prepared to become specific T-cells and B-cells to battle disease. It arrives at its maximal size before adolescence and, afterwards, begins to shrink and becomes obstructed with fat. As we age, we lose the ability to recover the thymus once it begins to debase.

Notwithstanding, as indicated by the proof, growth hormones can recover the thymus. Yet, it is incredibly diabetic. So clinical preliminaries for certain anti-diabetic medications, dehydroepiandrosterone (DHEA), and metformin are still going on. Metformin has a huge potential to safeguard against normal age-related illnesses like cancer and heart infections. Tests have been pulled off and they showed that fat stopped up in the thymus could be supplanted by restored thymus tissue.

Increased NAD levels can unlock the key to achieving youth, according to research led by Dr. David Sinclair's team. You can claim that if your body's NAD level is high, you can sprint for more than a minute without getting worn out or accumulating lactate.

Is it really possible to accomplish this? Well, it depends on where you are in your youth. Dr. Sinclair claimed that he and his colleagues could foster new compounds that would boost NAD levels. This NAD might be going about as an apparatus for speeding up reverse-ageing or, at the very least, a few side effects of being youthful.

This claim, believe it or not, is riddled with vagueness and squabbles. Some claim that NAD has a mending impact, but as per the ebb and flow research, it appears that NAD does not have a complete rejuvenating effect. Driving a sound way of life could urge you to battle infection, but increasing NAD levels have some sort of inadequacies when it comes to tissue regeneration. As a result, some experts are more sceptical about anti-ageing medicines' efficacy.

Another basic revelation has opened another room of reasoning. Yamanaka factors are exceptionally expressed in early-stage foundational microorganisms, and their over-articulation can instigate pluripotency in both mouse and human stem cells, showing that these elements control the signalling pathways fundamental for ES cell pluripotency.

Yamanaka factors by and large direct a formative signalling pathway made up of 16 formative signalling pathways, nine of which address prior obscure pathways in ES cells, including apoptosis and cell-cycle pathways. Yamanaka factors in mouse ES cells have additionally been considered. Curiously, this investigation likewise uncovered 16 formative signalling pathways, of which 14 cross-over with the ones uncovered by these studies, notwithstanding the way that the objective qualities and the signalling pathways controlled by every individual Yamanaka factor contrast altogether between these two datasets.

CHAPTER TWO

BEING YOUNG

If an elderly man is asked to describe his most exciting experience, he will most likely begin by saying, "When I was young..." and then proceed to describe his exciting experience. This is something we can never deny: they found the most entrancing portion of their lives to be living in their youth. But what's next? Isn't it true that they don't like this "old man" life? Well, no... However, if they restart with the same vehemence, it would be a spectacular opportunity for them. It'd be fantastic to reclaim that enticing vitality that each lady likes to succumb to. It would be truly wonderful to have the open door not to be hitched or to have the chance to go out and make anything we desired.

However, by and by, I also went over to an old man who confessed to feeling suicidal every so often. In any case, because of his child, he may yet get an opportunity to live once more. He still longed for the carefree days of his childhood. He appeared to have gotten back from his extended and agreeable get-away (a fun vacation). But he has lost his inspiration and is zeroing in just on carrying on with his life.

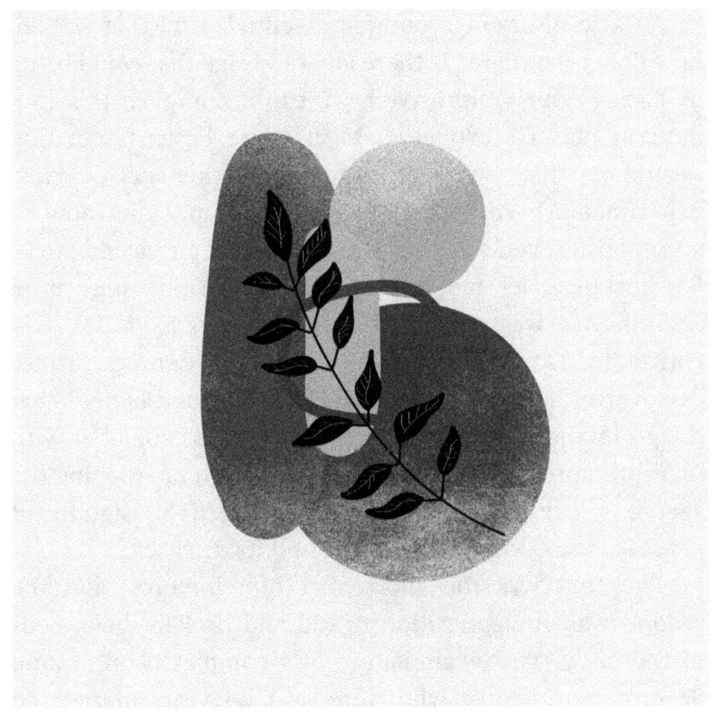

Our general public holds youth in high regard. Everybody loves to see those youthful, attractive celebs showing up on the screen. Every one of the ads for cosmetics is persuading us to purchase the substance with wizardry to assist us with looking less mature. Why are individuals so anxious to be youthful? What are the advantages of deferring the impacts of ageing? We can say that being youthful is generally lovely and cheering, and, surprisingly, later on, when we become older, I will think something similar: being youthful is the best thing that happens to each individual. When young, you are likely to be upbeat and urged to get on with your own life.

As a result, being young is essential. Isn't that so? So, how do we get there? Is there any beverage that could bring us back to our youth? Well, we can accomplish this in a number of ways. Nonetheless, it won't be as fascinating assuming that we get into it immediately.A few experiments have been done and are happening now to accomplish reverse ageing, which I have referenced before. For instance, let me inform you concerning one more analysis that was attempted by researchers from Tel Aviv University and the Shamir Medical Center, whose discoveries have been published in Aging magazine. What the group did was treat the cells in a tension chamber with high-pressure oxygen. They had the option of stopping the ageing process as well as reversing two significant processes associated with ageing and its diseases.

The first was the shortening of telomeres, and the second was an aggregation of old and broken down cells in the body. This examination was completed on around 35 grown-up people who were over 64 years of age and was important for the review. Every one of them was given hyperbaric oxygen treatments for an hour and a half daily, five times each week for quite a long time. In only three months, according to the review, the actual changes were identical to those of the members' bodies at the cell level 25 years earlier. Additionally, the subjects were found to have improved attention, information processing speed, and executive functions.

Moreover, we are likewise worried about what David Sinclair asserted. As per him, on the off chance that we pinch off a skin cell and develop it in a dish and put four Yamanaka factors on it, we can induce them to be changed into pluripotent stem cells. So, what exactly is a stem cell?

You can say it's the most youthful cell that has the ability to bring about a wide range of cells in our body, similar to how a photo frame can contain any type of A4-sized photo, certificates, and so on.

You can consider stem cells as blueprints that would lead to a wide range of cells in our body. As of now, you are adjusted to your matured cell. In the event that you attempt to induce them to rewind their biological clock, changing them over to the most youthful ones, you can't make them convert to stem cells. All things considered, your undeveloped cells are truly vulnerable to cancer. In any case, you can do a certain something.

You can make their signaling pathway end at one point where they become youthful again, but not so youthful that they lose their identity, which could turn out to be dangerous cells. However, it includes loads of blunders and needs exhaustive monitoring. We should be en route to let them know if the above process would work. OK, now ponder an incipient organism (embryo). Imagine a scenario in which we harm the sensory system of an embryo. It would absolutely recover within a brief timeframe. What if we damage the nervous system of an embryo? It would certainly grow back within a short period of time.

But in the case of adults, this is not hassle-free at all and often imparts failures owing to the complex process of development. You cannot grow them easily in adults. Regardless of whether you can do that, you should supplant them with new tissues, which is, in a real sense, inconceivable. Why? Since your body will expect them as unfamiliar materials and mount an insusceptible reaction against them, which would be considered malignancy.

The team of David Sinclair destroyed the optic nerves of some elderly mice. They discovered that their axons had died off, and the mice had gone blind. After that, they gave the mice three Yamanaka factors. They had experienced something spectacular after exposing those mice to those circumstances. The optic nerves began to regenerate, eventually returning all the way to the brain. We all know that as the developmental route begins, the fate of every gene in our body is sealed. Some have been turned off, while others have been turned on. This is maintained throughout our lives and is also employed to maintain the identity of our cells.

This allows all of our cells to function at their best. We can establish a cell's biological age by looking at its DNA methylation pattern. It may be conceivable to keep our biological age the same if we can keep our DNA methylation pattern the same or combine it with other factors in such a manner that genes display synonymous and optimum gene expression as previously. In this instance, after being exposed to Yamanaka factors, the blind mice appeared to be significantly younger. They repeated the experiment by inducing glaucoma, an age-related illness in which the retina of the eye is destroyed.

After being exposed to three Yamanaka factors, the mice were placed in front of a screen with moving lines. Those mice didn't just sit there looking after the treatment. After the treatment, those mice did not just sit there staring. They were really moving their heads in the direction of the lines, indicating that they had regained their vision and were beginning to notice the movement of the lines. But how did they regain their sight? Will this work in humans as well? For these more clinical trials are required. However, we might be able to reset or halt the age of a cell.

CHAPTER THREE

METFORMIN: A WONDER DRUG

To reset our age, we need to start somewhere. There are certainly some ways. Let's talk about them one by one. First, let's talk about some "druggish" ways. People who are suffering from diabetes probably know about metformin. It has been used for over 60 years to treat type II diabetes in the early stages because of its outstanding ability to decrease plasma glucose levels. Metformin is a widely used drug due to its safety and low cost. We know gluconeogenesis is dangerous for diabetic patients because it colossally enriches their blood sugar levels. It needs an appreciable amount of energy currency (6 ATPs are needed per molecule of glucose synthesized).

These ATP equivalents are given by the mitochondria to supply the hepatocytes' continual energy demand for gluconeogenesis. Metformin, which is positively charged, accumulates inside the mitochondrial inner membrane and inhibits complex I. As a result, ATP would not be produced in accordance with demand, reducing gluconeogenesis.

Late surveys have detailed the geroprotective impacts of biguanides, principally metformin, on account of their unrivalled wellbeing profile. As demonstrated before, metformin treatment improves insulin responsiveness, incites glycolysis, and smothers hepatic gluconeogenesis. There is some proof that metformin may likewise have cardioprotective impacts and add to the anticipation of certain types of human disease. This restorative profile of metformin upholds its utilization for age-related infections and life span.

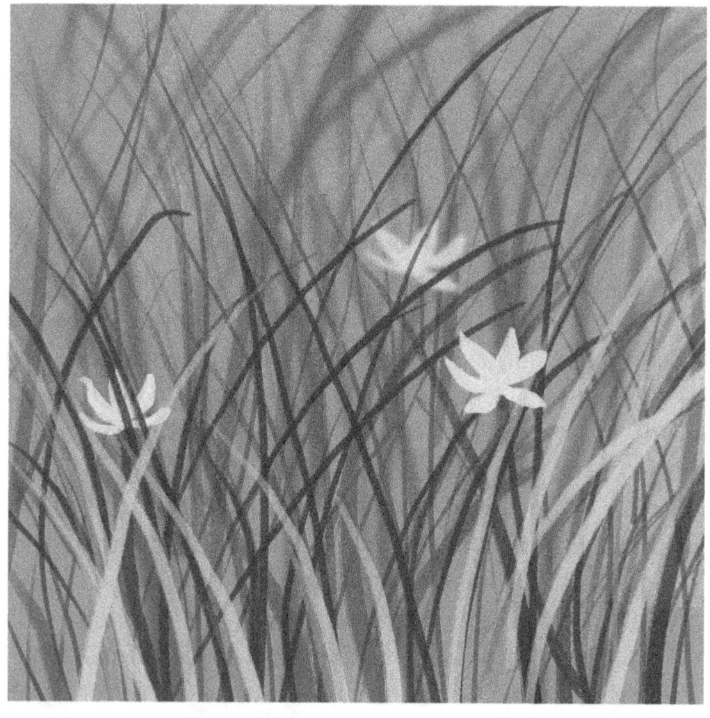

Of importance, many investigations have affirmed the constructive outcome of metformin on the life length of worms, flies, mice, and rodents. Also, diabetic and cardiovascular illness patients who are recommended metformin have expanded paces of endurance, and it was as of late suggested that metformin could extend life span by forestalling delicacy in more seasoned grown-ups with T2D. Persistent therapy with metformin among patients with diabetes could diminish the chance of mental deterioration and dementia and further develop endurance in a few sorts of diseases.

As indicated by late-distributed information in various creature models, metformin gives off an impression of being a promising up-and-comer as a daily existence-lengthening drug. This compound is, for the most part, very much endured, and its long history of clinical use makes it a significantly more appealing competitor. Additionally, metformin is more useful than some other anti-diabetic drugs in lessening age-related infections and further developing endurance in diabetic patients. Albeit the underlying outcomes are extremely confident, more work is expected to explain a few perspectives that actually stay hazy.

A considerable lot of these positive outcomes have been acquired utilizing dosages of metformin that surpass restorative levels in people. Besides, the methods of organization fluctuated among research groups, with the expansion of metformin either in drinking water or in the eating regimen. Although female mice were at first found to show a superior reaction to metformin supplementation, ongoing outcomes from our research centre demonstrated no orientation or stain contrasts in the activities of metformin.

Subsequently, to layout the atomic systems and pathways of maturing, it is important to explore potential chemical metformin collaborations in male and female creatures of fluctuating ages, as the period of beginning metformin treatment decides if an expansion in mean and greatest life expectancy happens. There are insufficient investigations to determine whether there are epigenetic/hereditary contrasts in metformin's impact on maturing, life length, and tumorigenesis. Since not all living beings examined appear to respond decidedly to metformin supplementation (e.g., flies and rodents), new methodologies with various conventions and trial plans would be critical to understanding how metformin may be a decent geroprotector all through phylogeny, remembering for people.

Metformin's history can be traced back many years. Galega officinalis, a medicinal spice popular in Europe, was known for improving stomach health and curing urinary problems and other ailments. Then, in 1918, a researcher discovered that one of its components, guanidine, might lower glucose levels. Guanidine-containing drugs, such as metformin and phenformin, were developed to treat diabetes. In any case, they become unfavourable as a result of the true side effects caused by phenformin and the release of insulin. Metformin was unearthed several years later and was licenced as a diabetes medication in Europe in the 1950s. Only after 1995 did the FDA approve its use in the United States. As a result of the legitimate adverse outcomes incurred by phenformin and the release of insulin, it has since become the most widely endorsed prescription.

We've known for a long time that metformin does more than just help diabetics lower their blood glucose levels. It also provides patients with cardiovascular benefits, such as a lower rate of cardiovascular morbidity and mortality. Furthermore, it every so often aids those with diabetes in losing unwanted pounds. Metformin may also offer medicinal benefits for those who do not have diabetes. Specialists have long prescribed it off-label, that is, for conditions other than those for which it is approved, such as: Prediabetes is characterised by elevated blood glucose levels that are not yet high enough to be diagnosed as diabetes.

In people with prediabetes, metformin may help to delay or perhaps prevent the onset of diabetes. Pregnant women may have elevated glucose levels, which return to normal following delivery. Metformin can help these women control their glucose levels throughout pregnancy. This issue will have a broad impact on young women whose ovaries support a variety of growth. Feminine abnormalities and troubles with richness are common. Despite the fact that the outcomes of clinical trials are mixed, metformin has been recommended for a long time for women with PCOS to help with female fertility, ripeness, and elevated glucose.

Antipsychotics are powerful medications used to treat mental illnesses such as schizophrenia. Massive weight gain is a common side effect. Metformin has been shown to reduce weight gain in some people who take these drugs. Analysts are also looking into metformin's ability to help people lose weight. It reduces the risk of illness in people who have type 2 diabetes. Malignant growths of the bosom, colon, and prostate are among them. Several studies have found that people with diabetes who take metformin have less mental decline and a slower rate of dementia, as well as a slower rate of stroke, than those who do not.

According to preliminary research, metformin may slow ageing and increase the body's insulin sensitivity, cancer prevention agent effects, and vein health. Because the vast majority of studies on metformin only involved people with diabetes or prediabetes, it's unclear whether these potential benefits are limited to those with those conditions, or whether people without diabetes could benefit as well.

Metformin has a very positive health profile. Queasiness, stomach distress, or bowel looseness are common side effects. However, these are usually mild. It would be interesting to see more true aftereffects. They include serious, adversely susceptible reactions as well as lactic acidosis, a lactic corrosive buildup in the circulatory system. Because the risk of this is increased in people who have a serious kidney infection, doctors will typically advise against using metformin for them. According to current diabetic guidelines, metformin is the first-line treatment for type 2 diabetes. It's not a big deal, and its potential consequences are well-known.

If you have diabetes and need metformin to help lower your blood sugar, the drug's other possible medical benefits are a wonderful - not harmful - side effect. What's more, what if you don't have diabetes at all? Indeed, its role in preventing or curing illnesses, and possibly, in any case, slowing down the maturation and expansion of the future, is even less evident. While the research thus far has been promising, we need more concrete evidence before recommending it to people who do not have diabetes.

Metformin, on the other hand, appears to be an excellent place to start for clinical professionals hoping to repurpose an existing pharmaceutical as a new wonder drug. Again, it is as yet under research. Clearly, tycoons are wagering on the opponent of anti-ageing research. As indicated by MIT Technology Review, Jeff Bezos, chief executive of Amazon, has put resources into Altos Labs, a strange new beginning up seeking after organic reconstructing to restore cells in the lab.

Anti-ageing strategies, in view of logical proof, intend to dial back the maturing system by forestalling or potentially postponing physiological decay and recovering lost practical capacities. A few methodologies incorporate supplementation with chemicals, including the development hormones dehydroepiandrosterone (DHEA), melatonin, and oestrogen, and wholesome enhancements that contain synthetic and natural antioxidants in cleaned structures or in plant extricates. Albeit a portion of these treatments have shown different clinical advantages in the treatment of the elderly, none truly tweaks the ageing process itself.

CHAPTER FOUR

RECENT WAYS TO LOOK YOUNGER

Cosmetic medicines for ageing are, in the best-case scenario, shallow and brief, and beauty care products are not lawfully permitted to influence or regulate basic cell and biochemical cycles. However, research has found different normal and engineered compounds that have a lot more prominent potential as gerontomodulatory particles than in their restricted use in beauty care products.

Another preventive methodology calls for adjusting our bodies to work on the fundamental sub-atomic and hereditary cycles of support and fix so they either work all the more proficiently or for longer. These purported "procedures for designed immaterial senescence" require updating utilitarian units of the body to the degree of genes, gene products, macromolecular interactions, sub-atomic milieu communications, etc.

Considering how little data and information we have at present about these connecting factors, it isn't clear how such a methodology would work in useful terms. Additionally, albeit piecemeal substitution of nonfunctional or harmed body parts leaves behind regular or engineered parts, it might give a brief answer to the issues related to ageing, but it doesn't balance the fundamental ageing process essentially.

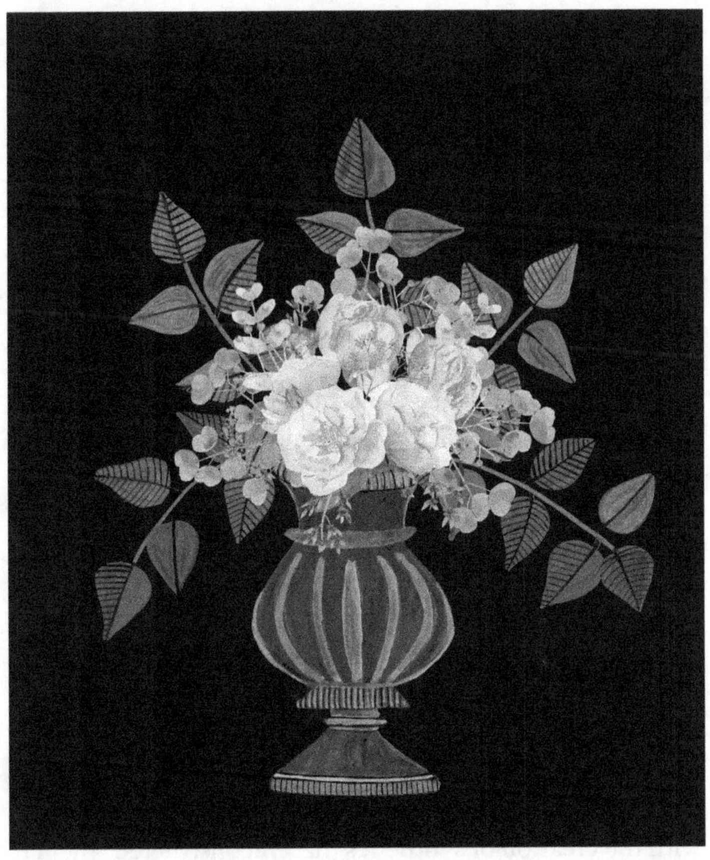

A more practical and promising way to deal with maturing mediation and anticipation is to utilize the body's inborn limits with regard to self-support and fix. It depends on perceptions that openness to low degrees of, if not unsafe, circumstances can animate homeodynamic versatile reactions that benefit individual cells as well as the entire organic entity. The hypothesis behind the methodology that low dosages of poisonous or hurtful substances have a defensive impact is known as hormesis.

Although the hormesis idea has been characterized in various settings like pharmacology and toxicology, hormesis in ageing is described by the gainful impacts that outcome from cell reactions to gentle rehashed stress. Uncovering cells and creatures to brief times of stress ought to hence dial back ageing since the hormetic reaction to pressure protects the living being against the stress as well as over-responds to eliminate other collected harm in cells and tissues.

The worldview of hormesis is working out, a movement that is both unpleasant and harmful because of the creation of free radicals, acids, stress chemicals, and cell and tissue breakage. Be that as it may, as an inducer of repair and upkeep processes, the hormetic impact of this demanding movement has a wide scope of wellbeing-advancing impacts.

Research from the Babraham Institute, a daily existence sciences research association in Cambridge, has likewise prompted the improvement of strategies that will fight off the sicknesses of old age by reestablishing the capacity of more seasoned cells and diminishing their natural age. In tests mimicking a skin wound, older cells were presented with the creation of synthetics that "reconstructed" them to act more like young cells and eliminate age-related changes. This has recently been accomplished, but the new work was finished in a much more limited time period—13 days compared to 50—and made the cells much more youthful.

The new strategy depends on the Nobel prize-winning method researchers use—which is enlivened by how old cells from guardians are transformed into the young tissues of an infant—to make stem cells. These are a sort of natural "clean canvas" without the markers of ageing. The Babraham research addresses a stage forward in light of the fact that this strategy doesn't totally eradicate the original cell. All things considered, the reconstructing system has ended partway, empowering scientists to find a harmony between making cells naturally more youthful while safeguarding their particular cell capacities.

The investigation gave promising indications that the restored cells would be better at mending wounds. The reconstructed cells delivered more collagen proteins, which assist in recuperating wounds, compared to cells that didn't go through the reinventing system. The scientists likewise saw that their technique reassuringly affected different qualities connected to progress in years of related illnesses and side effects. These include the APBA2 gene, which is related to Alzheimer's disease, and the MAF gene, which plays a part in the development of cataracts. The scientists said the component behind the reprogramming was not yet completely comprehended since it could cause malignant growth and should be additionally investigated before the discoveries can be applied to regenerative medication.

Presently, it is an ideal opportunity to be more youthful through conventional ways, or, we can say, to build NAD levels through regular ways. Numerous things make our skin age. A few things we can't make a meaningful difference with; others we can impact. One thing that can't be changed is the normal ageing process. It assumes a key part.

With time, we, as a whole, get apparent lines on our countenances. It is normal for our appearances to lose a portion of their youthful totality. We notice our skin becoming more slender and drier. Our genes generally control when these progressions happen. The clinical term for this kind of ageing is "ageing." We can impact one more sort of ageing that influences our skin. Our current circumstances and lifestyle decisions can make our skin age rashly. The clinical term for this sort of ageing is "extraneous ageing." By making a few preventive moves, we can slow the impact that this kind of maturing has on our skin.

The sun is a major contributor to our skin's premature ageing. Different things we do can cause our skin to age faster than it otherwise would have. Dermatologists provide the some advice to help their patients avoid premature skin ageing. How about we examine them individually in the following section.

CHAPTER FIVE

WAYS TO REJUVENATE

Safeguard your skin from the sun consistently. Whether going through a day on the ocean side or getting things done, sun insurance is fundamental. By seeking shade, wearing sun-protective clothing such as a lightweight and long-sleeved shirt, pants, a wide-overflowed cap, and UV-safe shades, and utilizing sunscreen with a broad range, SPF 30 (or higher), and is water-safe. You should apply sunscreen consistently to all skin that isn't covered by clothing. For more compelling insurance, search for a dress with a bright assurance factor (UPF) mark.

Assuming you smoke, quit. Smoking extraordinarily accelerates how rapidly skin ages. It causes wrinkles and a dull, colourless tone. Stay away from dull looks. Whenever you take a look, you contract the basic muscles. On the off chance that you contract similar muscles more than once in a long time, these lines become super durable. Wearing shades can assist with diminishing lines brought about by squinting. Eat a sound diet, even an eating routine. Discoveries from a couple of studies suggest that eating a lot of new products from the soil might assist in forestalling the harm that prompts untimely skin maturation. Discoveries from research concentrate additionally recommend that an eating routine containing loads of sugar or other refined starches can speed up ageing.

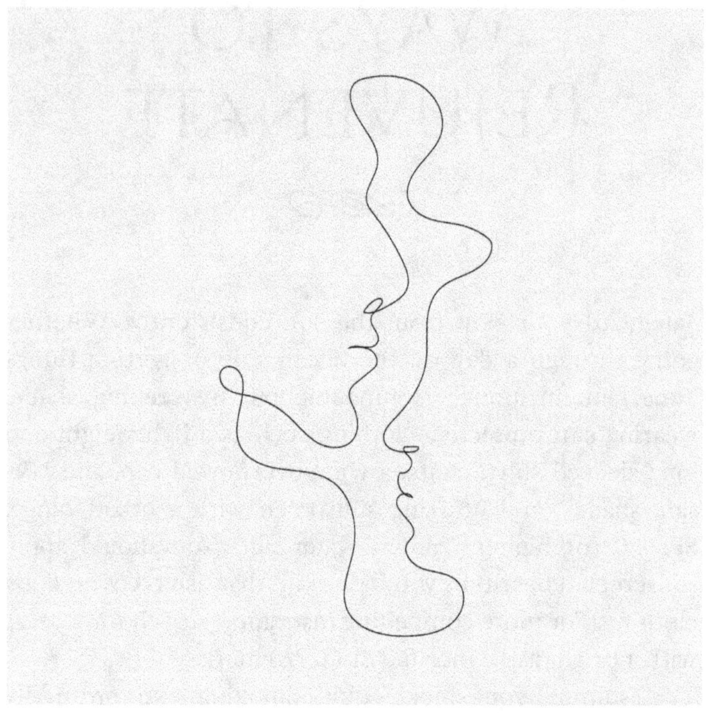

Practice most days of the week. Discoveries from a couple of studies recommend that moderate activity can further develop courses and lift the resistant framework. This, thus, may give the skin a more youthful appearance. Drink less liquor. Liquor is unpleasant on the skin. It dries out the skin and, on schedule, harms it. This can make us look more established. Purify your skin tenderly. Scouring your skin clean can disturb your skin. Bothering your skin speeds up skin ageing.

Delicate washing assists with eliminating contamination, cosmetics, and different substances without bothering your skin. Clean up twice a day and in the wake of perspiring intensely. Sweat, particularly while wearing a cap or cap, disturbs the skin, so you need to wash your skin quickly following perspiration. Apply a facial cream consistently. Cream traps water in our skin, giving it a more energetic appearance. Stop using healthy skincare products that sting or consume. Whenever your skin consumes or stings, it implies your skin is bothered. Disturbing your skin can make it look more established.

Perhaps the most straightforward method for returning to some time in the past is to make effective retinoids part of your skincare stockpile. While they can be bothersome to specific people with touchy skin, they can also give a genuine line of safeguard against wrinkles.

Try not to allow those little guilty pleasures to transform into additional pounds. Assuming that you do, you may very well end up looking more seasoned than you really are. Weight gain is additionally seen as maturing in a few regions. For instance, submental fat, which is situated underneath the jaw, essentially changes how the lower face is seen.

Zero in on a decent eating routine with a lot of lean protein and vegetables and keep away from sugar. Horrible eating routines that are high in sugar have been connected to cutting-edge glycation final results (AGEs), which cause kinks and loss of collagen and elastin.

Drinking a sufficient measure of water over the course of the day can assist in keeping your skin sound and young-looking. While how much water you want depends upon your size and activity level, tasting water over the course of the day and never allowing yourself to get parched is a decent rule.

Those late evenings you pulled in school are offering no courtesies to your skin. Truth be told, they could be the explanation for why you're looking somewhat worn out. Rest is quite possibly the main physiological interaction. While we are dozing, our bodies are fixing, detoxifying, and adjusting our chemicals. The coating of the GI plot is going over to guarantee your body can ingest every one of the supplements you are eating to keep your skin solid and cheerful. Sufficient rest further develops the course around the eyes, diminishing puffiness and dryness.

Do you figure you can avoid the shower after the exercise center? Reconsider. Cleaning up post-exercise can assist in keeping dead cleaning and other grime from subsiding into your pores, making them look bigger and, in this way, a definite indication of maturing. Clean up twice a day, particularly in the wake of perspiring intensely while working or working out.

Anti-ageing creams can be useful, but in the event that you need a significant change in the wellbeing and presence of your skin, begin with your food decisions and work outward.

Greasy fish and omega-3-rich seeds can assist your skin in making a fresh start, leaving you looking more youthful in a matter of seconds. Your body needs omega-3 fats found in endless amounts of fish oil, flaxseed, chia seeds, and pecans to be a critical part of cell films, and your body needs them to reestablish your skin cells. In this way, many individuals start eating better and, afterward, pass up these solid fats and end up with dry, flaky, or aggravated skin accordingly. Omega-3s aren't the best way to turn your well-being around in a rush; the 40 10-Second Health Fixes will make them look and feel improved in a moment.

Accumulating cancer prevention agents, whether through new products of the soil or supplementation, can make your skin better, and stronger, and make it look more youthful instantly. Silk pillowcases can assist your skin in withholding its normal dampness and decrease the presence of facial kinks.

Greasy fish isn't the best way to increase your admission of skin-firming omega-3s; pecans are additionally a decent choice for individuals who stay away from creature-based proteins. The omega-3 unsaturated fats in pecans assist in working on the versatility of the skin. Pecans additionally support collagen creation.

That hot shower might be unwinding, yet it very well may be draining your skin of fundamental dampness, making you look more seasoned simultaneously. Keep away from hot showers and showers; they'll dry out skin more than anything else.

All things considered, you don't need to fear solid oils in your food, and you don't need to fear them in your skincare schedule either. As a matter of fact, oil-based items can keep your skin hydrated and diminish your chances of harm. While you probably have no control over crying children on planes, gridlock, or waste vehicles outside your window at 5 a.m., attempting to de-stress as much and as frequently as possible can help you maintain a more youthful appearance. Getting sufficient rest, working out, and reflecting can all assist you with living with less pressure.

If you have any desire to stay away from pits and scarring that can make you look more established, quit picking at your skin immediately. Put an end to picking at those annoying breakouts and let them emerge all alone, or utilize regular items to assist with killing them. Any time you pick or pull at your skin, you're causing harm and making bother, scars, and, indeed, even kinks!

Candy won't help your skin, but that doesn't mean you can't appreciate something sweet occasionally. Truth be told, honey may very well assist in plumping your skin and keeping up with your imperishable look. This sweet treat is a characteristic humectant, meaning it draws in water. With regards to your skin, polishing off honey assists in drawing moisture from the mineral tissues to the outer layer of your skin, keeping it saturated, graceful, and drop-free.

L-ascorbic acid is additionally a significant piece of collagen, the protein that associates your cells together to form your skin's versatility and gives it structure. Ensure you are eating loads of citrus every day too, to get sufficient L-ascorbic acid so your body will make the collagen it requires to make a new skin framework. One serving of citrus natural products each day ought to get it done!

Notes

References I have used to babble my words:

- Anson RM, Guo Z, de Cabo R, Iyun T, Rios M, Hagepanos A, Ingram DK, Lane MA, Mattson MP (2003) Intermittent fasting dissociates beneficial effects of dietary restriction on glucose metabolism and neuronal resistance to injury from calorie intake. *Proc Natl Acad Sci USA* 100: 6216–6220.
- Bartke A, Chandrashekar V, Dominici F, Turyn D, Kinney B, Steger R, Kopchick JJ (2003) Insulin-like growth factor 1 (IGF-1) and aging: controversies and new insights. *Biogerontology* 4: 1–8.
- Beedholm R, Clark BF, Rattan SI (2004) Mild heat stress stimulates 20S proteasome and its 11S activator in human fibroblasts undergoing aging in vitro. *Cell Stress Chaperones* 9: 49–57.
- Bierhaus A et al. (2003) A mechanism converting psychosocial stress into mononuclear cell activation. *Proc Natl Acad Sci USA* 100: 1920–1925.
- Calabrese EJ, Baldwin LA (2000) Tales of two similar hypotheses: the rise and fall of chemical and radiation hormesis. *Hum Exp Toxicol* 19: 85–97.
- Carnes BA, Olshansky SJ, Grahn D (2003) Biological evidence for limits to the duration of life. *Biogerontology* 4: 31–45.
- de Grey AD (2000) Gerontologists and the media: the dangers of over-pessimism. *Biogerontology* 1: 369–370.
- Fonager J, Beedholm R, Clark BF, Rattan SI (2002) Mild stress-induced stimulation of heat shock protein synthesis and improved functional ability of human

fibroblasts undergoing aging *in vitro*. *Exp Gerontol* 37: 1223–1238.

- Gems D, Partridge L (2001) Insulin/IGF signalling and ageing: seeing the bigger picture. *Curr Opin Genet Dev* 11: 287–292.
- Hercus MJ, Loeschcke V, Rattan SI (2003) Lifespan extension of *Drosophila melanogaster* through hormesis by repeated mild heat stress. *Biogerontology* 4: 149–156.
- Hipkiss AR, Brownson C (2000) Carnosine reacts with protein carbonyl groups: another possible role for the anti-ageing peptide? *Biogerontology* 1: 217–223.
- Holliday R (1995) *Understanding Ageing*. Cambridge, UK: Cambridge University Press.
- Holliday R (2000) Ageing research in the next century. *Biogerontology* 1: 97–101.
- Hsiao G, Shen MY, Lin KH, Chou CY, Tzu NH, Lin CH, Chou DS, Chen TF, Sheu JR (2003) Inhibitory activity of kinetin on free radical formation of activated platelets *in vitro* and on thrombus formation *in vivo*. *Eur J Pharmacol* 465: 281–287.
- Kato K, Ito H, Kamei K, Iwamoto I (1998) Stimulation of the stress-induced expression of stress proteins by curcumin in cultured cells and in rat tissues in vivo. *Cell Stress Chaperones* 3: 152–160.
- Kirkwood TB (2002) Evolution of ageing. *Mech Ageing Dev* 123: 737–745.
- Le Bourg E (2005) Antioxidants and aging in human beings. In Rattan SIS (ed), *Aging Interventions and Therapies* pp85–107. World Scientific Publishers: Singapore.
- McFarland GA, Holliday R (1994) Retardation of the senescence of cultured human diploid fibroblasts by carnosine. *Exp Cell Res* 212: 167–175.

- McFarland GA, Holliday R (1999) Further evidence for the rejuvenating effects of the dipeptide L-carnosine on cultured human diploid fibroblasts. *Exp Gerontol* 34: 35–45.
- Minois N (2000) Longevity and aging: beneficial effects of exposure to mild stress. *Biogerontology* 1: 15–29.
- Olshansky SJ, Hayflick L, Carnes BA (2002) No truth to the fountain of youth. *Sci Amer* 286: 92–95.
- Padgett DA, Glaser R (2003) How stress influences the immune response. *Trends Immunol* 24: 444–448.
- Parsons PA (2000) Hormesis: an adaptive expectation with emphasis on ionizing radiation. *J Appl Toxicol* 20: 103–112.
- Partridge L (2001) Evolutionary theories of ageing applied to long-lived organisms. *Exp Gerontol* 36: 641–650.
- Raji NS, Surekha A, Rao KS (1998) Improved DNA-repair parameters in PHA stimulated peripheral blood lymphocytes of human subjects with low body mass index. *Mech Ageing Dev* 104: 133–148.
- Rattan SI (1995) Gerontogenes: real or virtual? *FASEB J* 9: 284–286.
- Rattan SI (1998) Repeated mild heat shock delays ageing in cultured human skin fibroblasts. *Biochem Mol Biol Int* 45: 753–759.
- Rattan SI (2000) Ageing, gerontogenes, and hormesis. *Indian J Exp Biol* 38: 1–5.
- Rattan SI (2001) Applying hormesis in aging research and therapy. *Hum Exp Toxicol* 20: 281–285.
- Rattan SI (2002) N^6-furfuryladenine (kinetin) as a potential anti-aging molecule. *J Anti-aging Med* 5: 113–116.
- Rattan SI (2003) Biology of aging and possibilities of

gerontomodulation. *Proc Indian Nat Sci Acad* B69: 157–164.

- Rattan SI (2004) Aging intervention, prevention, and therapy through hormesis. *J Gerontol A Biol Sci Med Sci* 59: 705–709.
- Slaugenhaupt SA, Mull J, Leyne M, Cuajungco MP, Gill SP, Hims MM, Quintero F, Axelrod FB, Gusella JF (2004) Rescue of a human mRNA splicing defect by the plant cytokinin kinetin. *Hum Mol Genet* 13: 429–436.
- Tatar M, Bartke A, Antebi A (2003) The endocrine regulation of aging by insulin-like signals. *Science* 299: 1346–1351.
- Verbeke P, Clark BF, Rattan SI (2001) Reduced levels of oxidized and glycoxidized proteins in human fibroblasts exposed to repeated mild heat shock during serial passaging in vitro. *Free Radic Biol Med* 31: 1593–1602.
- Verbeke P, Deries M, Clark BF, Rattan SI (2002) Hormetic action of mild heat stress decreases the inducibility of protein oxidation and glycoxidation in human fibroblasts. *Biogerontology* 3: 117–120.
- Vigh L et al. (1997) Bimoclomol: a nontoxic, hydroxylamine derivative with stress protein-inducing activity and cytoprotective effects. *Nat Med* 3: 1150–1154.
- Westerheide SD, Bosman JD, Mbadugha BN, Kawahara TL, Matsumoto G, Kim S, Gu W, Devlin JP, Silverman RB, Morimoto RI (2004) Celastrols as inducers of the heat shock response and cytoprotection. *J Biol Chem* 279: 56053–56060.
- Wood JG, Rogina B, Lavu S, Howitz K, Helfand SL, Tatar M, Sinclair D (2004) Sirtuin activators mimic caloric restricition and delay ageing in metazoans. *Nature* 430: 686–689.

- The article, Longevity and anti-aging research: 'Prime time for an impact on the globe', by The Harvard Gazette